T0197295

# TRANSFORMATION
# 28

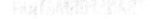

# TRANSFORMATION

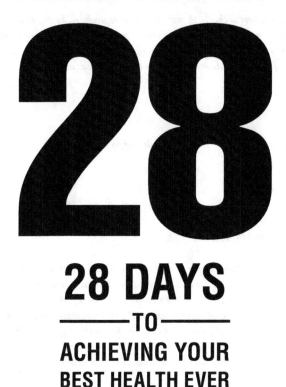

# 28

## 28 DAYS

——TO——

### ACHIEVING YOUR
### BEST HEALTH EVER

DR. NATHAN THOMPSON

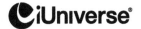
iUniverse®

# TRANSFORMATION 28
## 28 DAYS TO ACHIEVING YOUR BEST HEALTH EVER

iUniverse books may be ordered through booksellers or by contacting:

iUniverse
1663 Liberty Drive
Bloomington, IN 47403
www.iuniverse.com
1-800-Authors (1-800-288-4677)

Legal disclaimer: In view of the complex, individual nature of health and fitness problems, this book and the ideas, programs, procedures, and suggestions in it are not intended to replace the advice of trained medical professionals. All matters regarding one's health require medical supervision. A physician should be consulted prior to adopting any program described in this book. The contents of this book are based upon the opinions of the authors. The authors and publisher disclaim any liability arising directly from the use of the information contained in this book.

You should not undertake any diet/exercise regimen recommended in this book before consulting your personal physician. Neither the author nor the publisher shall be responsible or liable for any loss or damage allegedly arising as a consequence of your use or application of any information or suggestions contained in this book.

Any people depicted in stock imagery provided by Getty Images are models, and such images are being used for illustrative purposes only.
Certain stock imagery © Getty Images.

ISBN: 978-1-5320-5925-4 (sc)
ISBN: 978-1-5320-5924-7 (e)

Library of Congress Control Number: 2018911698

Print information available on the last page.

iUniverse rev. date: 10/24/2018

# CONTENTS

# FOREWORD

by Dr. Ben Lerner,
two-time *New York Times* best-selling author
and founder of Velocity Consulting and Coaching

I was really excited when Dr. Thompson informed me he had written a book on transformation in only twenty-eight days. The ability to change our lives and our bodies and even to transform might be the greatest gift bestowed upon us as a people. It is the inspiration of hope and the essence of the human spirit to know that you always have another chance, you can make a comeback, and a new you can be just around the corner.

I have written twenty books, two of which were *New York Times* best sellers. I have a bachelor's degree in nutrition and a master's in psychology, and I am a doctor of chiropractic. Additionally, I've been through every level of personal fitness training and life-coaching certification available, all to explore the straightest, most certain path to helping people reach their God-given potential. With all of that study and writing, I can tell you with certainty that if you follow Dr. Thompson's wisdom in the following pages, the idea of transforming in twenty-eight days is not simply hyperbole but a real possibility. It's something scientifically proven and that I have seen happen for thousands of people just like you.

Our tendency is to believe that life is pretty static. You inherit certain genes from your mom and dad and as a result are programmed into the person you are right now. The truth, however, is radically different. In fact, you are not stuck at all.

You contain approximately twenty thousand genes. That is a remarkably small amount, considering that a flea has about thirty thousand genes. Each of your twenty thousand genes can work with around two hundred proteins to create approximately four million different versions of you. This is great news for anyone who desires transformation in virtually any part of their life. If you are unsatisfied with your career, your emotional state, your health, or your physical body, dramatic change is very achievable.

You may already know someone who has experienced transformation in their life. A whole lot of people once were soft, out of shape, and worn out. They loved carbs, hated healthier foods, and would have rather attended a funeral than a fitness class. Yet after a period of just a few weeks or months, their attitudes about fitness, food, and bodies were metamorphosed. If someone else can do it, you can do it. Actually, if anyone else can do it, you can do it.

Recent gene research reveals that if you compare your genes to any other person, you will discover that 99.5 percent of the code is exactly the same. Therefore, very little has to do with luck, and it's not likely you are boxed into your current condition. If others can be fit, healthy, or make changes to their bodies, the odds are heavily in your favor that so can you. Our well-being is not based on a mere cosmic roll of the dice or a cruel, unfortunate genetic hand that we may have been dealt. No matter your past or your current situation, you have something to say about your future.

If you break down the word *transform*, you get "trans" and "form." *Trans*, like transport, is to take a journey—in this case, to take a journey into another shape or *form*. To further illustrate the possibilities that are out there for you, I have a couple of great stories about my patients who successfully made the journey.

Emily, a single mother, brought her sick young daughter to my clinic after she had gotten no results from any of the treatments or medications she previously had received. The concerned mother was a full-time hourly wage earner; the father was not in the picture or providing any financial support. While Emily was very diligent in following through with care, it was often with great difficulty that she kept up with the time and the costs involved.

After a few months, her daughter, once considered a lost cause by her doctors, became completely well. Not only did she transform, but her victory inspired Emily to go back to college and become a licensed general contractor. She eventually became an extremely wealthy and respected business leader in the community.

Another great story of transformation is Ron. Every male in his family had died of a heart attack in his fifties. When Ron turned fifty-two, he also had a heart attack. Thankfully, unlike the others, Ron lived. After this ordeal, he made a decision to honor the gift that life had handed him and get healthier every year for the rest of his life. Ron measured this by setting a new annual physical fitness record. He transformed his body and his life. When I met him, he was setting his new leg-press record at the gym we attended in Kissimmee, Florida, at the age of ninety-two.

You know you're a candidate for transformation when it seems impossible. In reality, few people find fitness easy or even possible to do. But remember: Transformation is a journey to a new form. Contained in this book is an achievable twenty-eight-day journey to transform your mind and body. If you trust the process, your attitude, your lifestyle, and what you think is possible for your future will change. For most, the change will be just the beginning of an ongoing new you. The unlimited you. The you that you were born to be.

Dr. Thompson is a longtime friend and colleague. He has gone through the transformation himself in his life, career, and physical body. The supermodel you see today was not the original Dr. Thompson that I met. He's not only the author of this book, but he's also walked the walk he's provided for you and that he has duplicated for many, many others.

I am personally praying for your transformation. As you transform, you will become empowered to be a courageous force for transformation in a dark and dying world. Together, we will make the world a better place to live, one renewed body and twenty-eight days at a time.

Live well.

Dr. Ben

# PREFACE

## The Straw That Broke the Camel's Back

If you've ever wondered why you tend to give up after a few days or weeks on the idea of living a lifestyle that will produce health, energy, and freedom, then this book was written for you. Many people wonder whether they have what it takes to radically change their lives and health for the better.

My answer is that you *do* have what it takes. In fact, everybody does. It's just a matter of reaching that final straw.

We all possess the power to change our lives and our lifestyles. Change in your life only happens when the pain of staying the same is greater than the pain that comes with change. My hope is that change happens in your life because you want to choose a better life, not because a crisis forced that change.

When I was growing up, I took a lot of pride in my fitness. I was the crazy kid running down the street with ankle weights, jumping rope in the driveway, and doing pull-ups in my backyard at night in the snow. I worked out to perform better in sports, and it helped me become a college athlete. But after college and graduate school, I didn't need to work out to perform, and that's when life happened. Opening a wellness office, working seventy hours a week, and having three kids in four years made me place my health on the back burner.

As a result, I slowly started to put on weight, lose my energy, experience poor sleep, and become stressed all the time. While I knew what was happening wasn't good for me (and I certainly wasn't happy with the direction I was going), I took comfort knowing that *one day* I was going to change. The problem was that *one day* never came. It became my excuse for *today's* destructive behavior. Something else was always more urgent or important—until something happened that changed my life forever.

It wasn't that I didn't fit into my pants anymore. It wasn't that my knees would creak like a seventy-year-old's going up the stairs. It wasn't even that I flunked my life insurance physical at thirty-two years of age. Do you know what my final straw was?

My dad was diagnosed with cancer.

After years of not taking care of himself and his *one day* never turning into *today*, it was time: he was forced to pay the consequences of his actions, not his good intentions. With his diagnosis, I knew that if I didn't change, I would end up just like him, and I didn't want my kids to experience the same level of worry and fear that I experienced about my dad. I had become so tired and frustrated about the direction of my health that absolutely nothing was going to stop me from doing what I needed to do to reclaim my health and take ownership of my future. I reached my final straw.

Do you know what happened? In an instant, I shifted my mind-set from one of excuses to one of massive action. Within a few short weeks I lost twenty-three pounds and got in the best shape of my life, and I have continued to become even better, years after that life-changing decision.

I'm busier than ever before, but that doesn't deter me. I've made my health and fitness a top priority in my life, and I don't regret it one bit.

I want you to know that I'm no better than you and I don't possess more talents, gifts, or willpower than you do. I know that if I can do it, you can do it too.

But my question for you is this: What will be *your* final straw?

With my transformation came a burden, the burden of helping people who were just like me, struggling with their weight, their energy, and a lack of direction. I began a journey of learning everything I could about nutrition, how to overcome food addictions, and the best way to exercise in the shortest amount of time. That led me to pursue advanced certifications in nutrition and exercise methodology. The real art was knowing not just the information but how to package and present it to people in a way that was easy to understand and doable for anybody.

I started to do challenges to help people change their nutrition and fitness over twenty-eight days using simple nutrition strategies and fun workouts in a group setting, as well as helping people discover the right mental framework in which to have massive success. Over the course of a few years, people started to contact me for information regarding this challenge their friends went through. And the inspiration to write a book about it was born.

Chances are you've already read a book about nutrition and fitness. I can assure you this book is different. This approach is unconventional. But if you're reading this book, convention likely has not worked for you. It's time for a different approach.

You're on your way to learning why you gain weight; why you crave certain foods; why you might have blood sugar, blood pressure, and/or cholesterol issues; why you have chronic pain; and why your exercise (or lack of it) is sabotaging your health. Not only that; you'll learn how to develop the right mind-set and plan that will help you become the best version of yourself.

If you follow what's in this book, I know that transformation will happen over the next twenty-eight days, not only physically but mentally as well.

Look at yourself in the mirror. Say goodbye to your former self and hello to the brand-new you! Thousands of others have joined me on the mountaintop by following the contents of this book. I can't wait to see you there too.

I believe in you.

Dr. Nathan Thompson

# ACKNOWLEDGMENTS

There are many people to thank who have given me the strength and courage to write a book. I'll admit there's always been that voice in the back of my mind that wondered if I was good enough or smart enough or if people would even listen. I'd be remiss not to mention a few people who have helped shape me and given me the motivation to make a difference in people's lives.

Mom and Dad, thank you for always demanding excellence in everything. You taught me that how I do anything is how I'll do everything. I remember the times vividly when you looked at me in the eye and said, "I believe in you!"

Rick Tollefson, thank you for being my favorite coach growing up. I learned so much from you about effort and humility. I consider you not only a mentor and tremendous visionary but also a friend. Thank you for your support in my vision.

Dr. Ben Lerner, thank you for providing me the vision on how to make my profession my mission. Your direction has always inspired me to never settle for something small.

Greg Glassman, thank you for being a visionary and pioneer in the field of health and fitness. Your system of fitness, known as CrossFit©, has helped me gain the fitness and confidence that I lacked for years. You have helped me discover that my best years of health are ahead of me and not a thing of the past. Thank you for being relentless in your passion to help people like me.

And finally, many thanks to my wife, Barb, and to my Exemplify coaches and staff for being so gracious and stepping up your efforts to give me the freedom to write a book while still being in full-time practice and maintaining two amazing fitness centers, where lives are transformed every day.

# CHAPTER 1

# The Magic Is in the Mind-Set

Have you ever started a new diet or fitness routine and been convinced that this new strategy was your ticket to a brand-new life? Have you quit this new diet and fitness routine within a few days, few weeks, or a few months?

If this is you, you're not alone. I had started and stopped too many times to count until I discovered the reason why.

The reason why so many people fail to make a permanent change to their lifestyle is that they have convinced themselves that transformation happens by finding the right strategy. Watch an hour of prime-time television, and you'll see commercials for newfangled ideas or contraptions making promises of rock-hard abs, buns of steel, and shapely hips. And we fall for it—hook, line, and sinker.

After a few days, we get bored with the strategy, give up, and feel like a failure. Each time this happens, it becomes harder to convince ourselves that true transformation can actually happen, and finally we became resolved to the idea that having an amazing body, abundant energy, and Olympic-level fitness was never meant to be.

But what if instead of placing your hope in the strategy, you first pursued the right mind-set? What if you could develop the mental makeup of someone who refuses to quit? If you could reframe your brain and learn to change the way you think, even a mediocre strategy would be better than a great strategy with a poor mind-set.

It's only after changing your mind-set does the strategy even matter. And I have a strategy that works 100 percent of the time, as long as you are willing to put in the work and not give up.

If you've failed at the whole diet-and-exercise routine, I have a question for you: *Why* did you fail?

You may have a lot of different reasons:

- I haven't found the right plan.
- I've been too busy.
- I'm too old.
- It's too hard.
- I have arthritis.
- I have bad genes.

Unfortunately, these reasons aren't valid. They're just rational lies you tell yourself that keep you from taking massive action and changing your life. When it's all said and done, your health accepts only action, not intentions or excuses. But the great news is that you can change, and that change is entirely up to you and not your circumstances.

*Remember: You can have results or reasons but not both.*

# CHAPTER 2

# Fat-Loss Myths and Truths

Now that you're on your way to discovering the right mind-set, you need the right plan. You can have the noblest of intentions to change, but without the right plan, you'll never get the results you want.

Here's one of the biggest myths regarding fat loss and fitness:

> *Fat-Loss Myth*: Fat loss is about calories in and calories
> out, food deprivation, and hours of exercise.

In reality, a calorie is not just a calorie. The food that contains the calories and what it does to your hormones makes all the difference. And it's not about exercising to burn more calories. It's about exercising to produce a hormone response in order to burn fat and build muscle. How many calories you burn during exercise doesn't matter as much as the hormone response you get *after* you're done exercising.

> *Fat-Loss Truth*: Fat loss is actually about regulating hormones,
> such as insulin and human growth hormone, by eating the right
> types of foods and by incorporating the right type of fitness.

You'll find that if you can get your hormones under control by eating and exercising according to how your body was designed to function, you can achieve the results you've always wanted and dramatically shift your health, function, and vitality.

A note of caution: Don't become *that guy* (or girl) who thinks that everything is black and white. Rarely are things ever that cut and dry, especially when it comes to nutrition and fitness. We desire things to be black and white. We also like to think of nutrition and fitness ideas as a series of commandments. I've worked with thousands of patients on nutrition and fitness, and one of the first questions I get is, "Is [insert a food or exercise program] good or bad?"

As you read this book, it can be very easy to fall into the black-and-white nutrition and fitness trap. To prevent this, I want you to remember that very rarely is a food or a form of exercise all bad. Everyone has different performance and health goals, so it's best to look at it as a continuum.

All Bad—Pretty Bad—It Depends—Pretty Good—All Good

For example, let's say I've been stranded on a deserted island with no food for thirty days. One day, you come along in a boat and discover me at the point of starvation. In your boat is a double cheeseburger, French fries, and a supersized sugary beverage, which you offer me (I won't ask why it's in your boat!). At that point, do you think I would say, "No thanks. I heard this food isn't good for my health"?

Of course not.

Although it's not going to be the healthiest for me, I'll gladly eat that food because it still has some nutrients to keep me alive. But listen—if you're reading this book, you're probably not suffering from starvation. In fact, there's a good chance that you're actually overfed and undernourished.

So, if you ever find yourself stranded on a deserted island, I won't cast a scornful eye if you eat that double cheeseburger to keep you alive.

# CHAPTER 3

# World-Class Nutrition in Twenty-Five Words

My goal is to make it easier, not harder, for you to understand nutrition. While nutrition is a relatively new and complex science, it can be broken down into something simple and easy to understand. Consider these twenty-five words, adapted from Greg Glassman, founder of CrossFit:

Eat meat and vegetables, nuts and seeds, some fruit, little starch, and no sugar. Keep intake to levels that support exercise but not body fat.

Over the next few chapters, I'll answer the following questions:

- Why only a little starch and no sugar?
- Why only some fruit?
- What types of meat and vegetables?
- What types of nuts and seeds?
- How should they be prepared?

Let's begin by looking at the big picture. All food is broken down into three main macronutrients and their functions:

1. Carbohydrates or sugar—energy
2. Protein—repair

3.  Fat—protection, hormone function, storage of fat-soluble vitamins, and energy

I'll also break down the best and worst of each kind of macronutrient to help you get your nutrition back on track.

# CHAPTER 4

# Why It's Best to Avoid Added Sugar, Starch, and Grains and Limit Fruit

There are many reasons why you should avoid added sugar, starch, and grains and limit fruit, and I want to go over my top five reasons. For simplicity's sake, let's define sugar, grains, and fruit by what they turn into when digested: sugar.

**Reason 1:** Added sugar is the number one cause of obesity.

According to the United States Department of Agriculture, the average American consumes almost seventy-five pounds of added sugar per year. As added sugar consumption has increased, so has obesity, and we have a big problem with obesity-related illness today.

Recent studies published in the *Journal of the American Medical Association* (*JAMA*) show that 35 percent of American men, 40 percent of women, and 17 percent of children and adolescents are obese, with a body mass index (BMI) of 30 or higher.

And those numbers are only getting worse. It is estimated that half of all American adults will be obese by 2030, which is costing us a *lot* of money.[1]

The Robert Wood Johnson Foundation predicts that annual economic productivity lost due to obesity will be a staggering $580 billion by 2030, unless the current situation changes. That's almost $2,000 lost for every man, woman, and child in the United States.[2]

Being overweight is not only unhealthy; it's downright expensive!

*Why does sugar cause weight gain and obesity?*

When it comes to using sugar for energy, your body can handle only a small amount of sugar at one time. Then, whatever your body doesn't need for immediate energy goes straight into storage. First it stores that sugar in the muscles and liver in a form known as glycogen. Once the liver and muscles reach their storage capacity, the liver turns sugar into triglycerides (free fat in the blood), where it is then stored in your fat cells. The hormone responsible for this is called insulin.

**Reason 2:** Added sugar is your fast track toward prediabetes and type 2 diabetes.

Research shows that once you reach the level where 18 percent of your daily calories comes from added sugar, there's a twofold increase in metabolic harm that promotes prediabetes and diabetes.[3]

Because of our poor eating habits, prediabetes and diabetes are the fastest-growing chronic injuries (not illnesses) among adults *and* children today.[4]

> Type 2 diabetes is an injury, not an illness. Once you remove what's *causing* the injury, you can allow the body to heal.

Once you're diagnosed with type 2 diabetes, you've already been sick for years. The conventional medical approach is to diagnose you with a disease once you have it. Wouldn't you rather know that you're on your way toward developing diabetes *before* you have it?

Here's a simplified version of how you develop type 2 diabetes and everything that goes wrong with the traditional management of it.

Let's say you decide to start smoking. At first, the nicotine from one cigarette per day will give you a buzz. But soon, you'll need two cigarettes a day for the same buzz, and then four, and then a whole pack. In a few years, you'll notice that smoking a whole pack of cigarettes does nothing to create that same buzz you had just a few years ago. This concerns you, so you go to your primary care doctor to remedy the situation. After careful analysis and testing, your doctor comes back with the definitive diagnosis.

"I have good news and bad news," your doctor says. "The bad news is that you're not responding to nicotine anymore; it's called nicotine resistance. The good news is that if you increase to four packs a day, it will start to give you a buzz in no time."

That sounds crazy, right? But the same thing happens with the hormone insulin.

Any time you consume a food that turns to sugar, it enters your bloodstream as glucose and raises your blood sugar. The brain senses this increase in blood sugar and sends a message to your pancreas to release insulin. Once insulin is released into the bloodstream, it attaches to the receptors on the various cells in your body that open channels to allow glucose to enter the cell to be used as energy. The glucose that's not used as energy will get stored as glycogen in the liver and muscles. But the body can store only a small amount (about 600 grams). Anything more than that gets stored as fat.

And there's no limit to how much fat you can store!

The problem arises when you are constantly bombarding the cells with insulin. As with any hormone or drug, when it's present in large amounts, the cells begin to adapt by decreasing the number of receptors on the cell, in turn decreasing your sensitivity to it. The less sensitive you are to insulin, the more you'll need to make in order to elicit the same response and the more difficulty you will have keeping your blood sugar balanced.

When your doctor finally discovers a blood sugar problem, the medical standard of care requires you to go on a drug that will stimulate the production of more insulin.

While the pancreas can keep up with the increased workload for a little while and push your blood sugar levels down, eventually it will tire out, and that's when things get really bad. With smoking, the way to resensitize your cells to nicotine is to withdraw yourself from nicotine. And the way to resensitize your cells to insulin is not to add more insulin but to withdraw yourself from the hormone. The way to decrease this hormone naturally is to withdraw from foods that spike your blood sugar and cause a massive dump of insulin into the body.

### Warning Signs That You Have a Problem with Insulin Right Now

- You have to eat sugar every few hours to avoid feeling fatigued.
- You experience "brain fog" if you don't have enough sugar throughout your day.
- You experience mood swings and irritability if you don't have sugar throughout your day.
- You feel you have to eat every few hours in order to avoid being hungry.

Is this you? Don't worry. I'll go over the plan you can utilize to withdraw from sugar. In a few days or weeks, you can feel energized, feel full all day, decrease your pain levels, and increase your mental clarity. I'll also describe how you will feel during this process and what to monitor so that you can stay the course and have massive success.

**Reason 3:** Added sugar causes inflammation in the body, contributing to arthritis, pain, high blood pressure, and even high cholesterol.

A 2014 study in the *Journal of the American Medical Association* found those who consumed the most sugar—about 25 percent of their daily calories—were twice as likely to die from heart disease as those who limited their sugar intake to 7 percent of their total calories.[5]

The cause of this is *inflammation*—the link to nearly all disease.

When you get a cut on your skin, you've probably noticed that it gets red, swollen, painful, and hot. This is a normal, innate inflammatory response that tissues require for healing. That inflammation signals the body to begin laying down scar tissue to heal the wound.

Inflammation is a great thing, except when it never ends.

There's little doubt that sugar increases inflammation in the body, but it's not the acute inflammation that you normally see in a cut or with a sprained ankle. Instead, it's a chronic, low-grade type of inflammation that not only damages your joints, leading to arthritis and increased pain, but also damages your arteries.

When chronic inflammation is present in your arteries, they too get red, swollen, and hot (but not painful because they don't have pain receptors). When the blood vessels swell, their diameters gets smaller. When the diameters gets smaller, the heart has to work harder to get blood, nutrients, and oxygen to the tissues ... and that's called high blood pressure.

Cholesterol is *not* the villain. You just need to stop beating up your arteries.

Any time there's inflammation, there has to be healing, and guess what the body uses to heal the damage in your arteries? You guessed it: cholesterol. To heal the damage inflammation inflicts on your arteries, cholesterol must be laid down within the arteries to heal and repair them. In short, more inflammation means your liver needs to produce more cholesterol, and that's why your cholesterol levels go up.

In reality, the innate response of increasing blood pressure and cholesterol is the right response at the right time. While this process helps to save your life in the short term, this long-term adaptation leads to hardening of the arteries and cardiovascular disease.

The problem is not your high blood pressure or cholesterol. The problem is inflammation. Get to the cause of high blood pressure and cholesterol by lowering inflammation.

### *Should I be taking a cholesterol-lowering drug?*

While I can't tell you what to do, I can share research on the effectiveness of cholesterol-lowering drugs.

You have between a 0.4 and 1 percent chance of benefitting from a cholesterol-lowering drug, but you have a 15–20 percent chance of developing one the following side effects:

- headache
- constipation
- diarrhea
- gas
- stomach pain
- skin rashes
- muscle and joint pain
- muscle wasting
- liver failure
- dementia
- depression

This research was published in 2008 by John Carey in *BusinessWeek* magazine, based on his analysis of the effectiveness of cholesterol-lowering drugs.[6]

**Reason 4:** Added sugar and grains fuel cancer.

Eating sugar doesn't cause cancer. If it did, everyone who eats a lot of sugar would get cancer. Cancer is a multifactorial disease, but sugar can certainly fuel it. Cancer cells have a completely different metabolic makeup than a normal, healthy cell. In fact, cancer cells have approximately ten times more receptors for insulin than a normal cell. Therefore, the preferred fuel for cancer cells is sugar (glucose).

"But my doctor said what I eat has no relation to cancer!"

Do you know how doctors identify whether cancer has spread to other parts of the body? They use what's called a PET scan. Known as positron emission tomography (PET), this test is a nuclear imaging technique that creates detailed, computerized pictures of organs and tissues inside the body. A PET scan reveals how the body is functioning and uncovers areas of abnormal metabolic activity.

In preparation for a PET scan, a patient is first injected with a glucose (sugar) solution that contains a very small amount of radioactive material. This substance is absorbed by the particular organs or tissues being examined. The PET scanner is then able to "see" damaged or cancerous cells where the glucose is being taken up (cancer cells often use more glucose than normal cells) and the rate at which the tumor is using the glucose (which can help determine the tumor grade).

> *Read that again*: Doctors use *sugar* to detect *where*
> the cancer is and how *aggressive* it is.

Kind of makes you wonder, doesn't it?

**Reason 5:** Added sugar is addictive—even more addictive than cocaine!

Added sugars and grains are far more addictive than cocaine, one of the most addictive, harmful substances available to us. An astonishing

94 percent of rats who were allowed to choose between sugar water and cocaine chose sugar. Even rats who were addicted to cocaine quickly switched their preference to sugar, once it was offered as a choice.[7]

Our sugar-rich standard American diet generates a surge in a neurochemical in the brain called dopamine, which is widely known as the neurochemical responsible for pleasure and motivation. But substances like cocaine, heroin, nicotine, and other drugs produce this excessive reward signal in the brain as well. This signal then has the potential to override normal self-control mechanisms and thus leads to addiction.

So let me ask you … Is sugar your drug of choice?

While you may take comfort in the fact that you don't drink or smoke, chances are you probably have a different addiction—an addiction to sugar. Similar to the alcoholic who craves alcohol, what do you think your brain will tell you when you crave sugar? It will tell you that you're hungry, and you will reach for that next dose of sugar.

The next time you feel hungry, ask yourself, "Is this physical hunger, or is it psychological hunger?" If you can reach down and grab more than an inch of fat around your belly or thighs, you already know the answer. That hunger is all in your head.

*My first introduction to the addictive nature of sugar went like this:*

Several years ago, I headed up a huge potluck dinner at my church. I thought it would be a wonderful idea to teach people how to cook healthy food without using all the sugar, additives, and damaging fats that are in foods normally seen at a church potluck. I thought everyone would *love* my innovative idea!

I believe I received seven death threats from church members. Okay, not really, but the responses I received were hardly positive:

"You're taking away my bread and cookies? How dare you!"

"I look forward to eating whatever I want on Sundays!"

"I was going to bring friends to church that day, but now we're going out for pizza instead because if we come to the potluck, they won't want to ever come back to this church!"

If food generates a strong emotional response, you probably are addicted to it.

By the way, the potluck went over really well, and several people apologized afterward because they were astounded how good *real* food actually could taste.

*Why hasn't my doctor taught me any of this?*

I believe doctors truly want to help you. While I can't speak for every doctor, I can certainly offer some possible explanations:

- Your doctor was trained in the diagnosis and management of disease through medications and surgery and received very little training in the field of nutrition or exercise science in school.

- Your doctor must follow a standard of care. A standard of care is a treatment that is accepted by medical experts as a proper treatment for a certain type of disease and that is widely used by health care professionals. Many times, the standard of care calls for drugs or surgery, not lifestyle modification.

- Your doctor may know how to help you, but it's not reimbursable through insurance or not profitable enough. Or maybe your doctor believes you won't follow through because you'll think it's too hard.

So are all carbs bad, then?

Absolutely not! You do need carbohydrates to function, but you don't need as many as you think. But there are great carbohydrates, okay carbohydrates, and carbohydrates to avoid at all costs. The difference between these types of carbohydrates is the insulin response they cause.

## The Best Types of Carbohydrates

- vegetables

What's the difference between boogers and broccoli?
Kids don't eat broccoli.

Funny (or not so funny) jokes aside, it seems that many adults don't like to eat broccoli or vegetables either as their preferred source of carbohydrates (and hopefully don't prefer boogers!).

Vegetables are always best because they are full of fiber, vitamins, and minerals needed for healthy cellular function, and they have the lowest insulin response. Vegetables are best when eaten raw, lightly steamed, or sautéed with coconut oil. The best vegetables are those that contain sulforaphane, which gives them a slightly pungent odor (like broccoli).

*Getting your daily vegetables and greens just got easier.*

If you find it hard to get your six to nine servings of vegetables per day, then have no fear. A secret I've used for years—for me and for my kids—is to consume an organic-greens powder. This powder contains some of the top superfoods available today, and they are full of antioxidants. I mix an organic-greens powder with a smoothie or in water every day. For more information on the greens powder I recommend, visit *Transformation28.net*.

- berries, Granny Smith apples, and grapefruit

These fruits are the lowest in sugar and are higher in fiber, so they won't impact your blood sugar and insulin levels like other fruits. However, these fruits should be consumed in moderation because they still contain some sugar.

You may be thinking, *Isn't fruit natural?* Absolutely! But chances are you've been doing some very unnatural things when it comes to fueling your body, and the resulting weight gain, chronic pain, and/or hormone issues are not natural. You'll have to avoid them for a while until your hormones and inflammatory levels normalize.

The following carbs can be good or bad, depending on your current health and fitness goals:

➤ all fruits other than berries, Granny Smith apples, and grapefruit
➤ sweet potatoes
➤ legumes: peas, beans, and lentils
➤ sprouted grains

These carbs can be utilized in moderation for those who perform daily high-intensity exercise or endurance-type exercise, and/or for those who have achieved their weight-loss goals and healthy blood work. Those who have issues with weight gain, insulin resistance, type 2 diabetes, autoimmune conditions, leaky-gut syndrome, cancer, blood pressure, and/or cholesterol need to avoid them. Over time, you may be able to reintroduce these foods in moderation.

**Carbs to Always Avoid**

• refined wheat flour

Refined wheat flour is nothing more than sugar. It contains only the endosperm of the grain, which contains the carbohydrates and a small amount of protein, known as gluten. Refined wheat flour is devoid of the bran and the germ, which contain the vitamins, minerals, fat, and fiber. Instead of baking with wheat flour, try coconut or almond flour instead.

• table sugar

Also known as sucrose, this finely ground white powder is more addictive than another addictive, finely ground white powder—cocaine.

- anything ending in *-ose* and sugar's different aliases

Sugar has a lot of different names, and people are starting to wise up. However, food manufacturers are working day and night to stay one step ahead by giving sugar even more names. Below is a list of the different names for sugar. Take a deep breath; it's a long one!

## The Different Names of Sugar

| | | | |
|---|---|---|---|
| agave nectar | corn sweetener | glucose solids | muscovado |
| barbados sugar | corn syrup | golden sugar | palm sugar |
| barley malt syrup | corn syrup solids | golden syrup | panocha |
| beet sugar | date sugar | grape sugar | powdered sugar |
| brown sugar | dehydrated cane juice | high-fructose corn syrup | raw sugar |
| buttered syrup | demerara sugar | honey | refiner's syrup |
| cane juice | dextrin | icing sugar | rice syrup |
| cane juice crystals | dextrose | invert sugar | saccharose |
| cane sugar | evaporated cane juice | malt syrup | sorghum syrup |
| caramel | free-flowing brown sugar | maltodextrin | sucrose |
| carob syrup | fructose | maltol | sugar (granulated) |
| castor sugar | fruit juice | maltose | syrup |
| coconut palm sugar | fruit juice concentrate | mannose | treacle |
| coconut sugar | glucose | maple syrup | turbinado sugar |
| | | molasses | yellow sugar |

- white potatoes and white rice

Composed almost entirely of starches (long chains of sugars), white potatoes and white rice raise your blood sugar quickly, which results in a large increase in insulin. Although there are some vitamins and minerals in these foods, you can easily get them from other sources that are lower in sugar.

- high-fructose corn syrup

Commonly found in sweetened beverages like soda and fruit juice, high-fructose corn syrup is perhaps the worst type of sugar for your health.[8] Refined fructose is metabolized much like alcohol, causing damage to your liver and metabolic dysfunction in the same way that ethanol and other toxins do. Not only that, but high-fructose corn syrup is more readily metabolized into fat than any other form of sugar.

- condiments and salad dressings

Always look at the label when purchasing packaged food. You can fall off track on your nutrition journey by adding things like ketchup and salad dressings to your nutrition. These foods often have a lot of added sugar. It's best to use these sparingly and to use healthy oils and vinegar when having any type of salad.

*Are you allergic to gluten, or are you just allergic to poison?*

Gluten is the protein found in wheat, rye, barley, spelt, and a few other closely related grains. Almost all processed food contains gluten for one reason or another: thickening, flavor, as a binder, or as a major ingredient in pizza, pasta, cakes, cookies, and bread, to name a few.

The gluten-free movement has gained considerable traction over the past few years. There are people who are truly gluten-intolerant and find tremendous benefit from removing gluten from their diet. But why is it that so many people have seemingly become allergic to gluten?

After all, our genetics can't change that much over a few years, which makes it impossible that everyone suddenly has a genetic intolerance to gluten.

Maybe it's not a gluten intolerance. Maybe it's a reaction to glyphosate.

Glyphosate is the main herbicide in the weed killer Roundup, which is sprayed on many crops today to reduce the undesirable weeds in agricultural fields. Glyphosate is toxic to most plants, including corn and soybeans, so these crops have to be genetically modified in order to be resistant to this popular herbicide, and glyphosate has the potential to end up in you.

Although wheat has yet to be genetically modified, it is still sprayed with glyphosate just prior to harvest in order to completely kill the wheat and speed up the drying process. This preharvest spraying means that the level of glyphosate on the wheat is far higher than in other genetically modified crops, like corn or soybeans.

This toxin may be what's wreaking havoc on your digestive and immune systems. Did I also mention that glyphosate was classified as a probable carcinogen by the World Health Organization in 2015?[9]

# CHAPTER 5

# The Not-So-Sweet Truth about Artificial Sweeteners

At this point, you might be thinking, *This is great! I still get to eat and drink my diet products.*

Not so fast.

Let me ask you two questions:

1. Have you ever seen a really healthy person drinking or eating "diet" products?
2. Have you ever wondered why?

*Artificial sweeteners cause "metabolic confusion."*

One of the reasons why artificial sweeteners do not help you lose weight is that your body is not fooled by a sweet taste without the accompanying calories.

When you eat something sweet, like chocolate, your brain releases dopamine, which activates your brain's reward center. The appetite-regulating hormone leptin is also released, which eventually informs your brain that you are full, once a certain number of calories have been ingested.

However, when you consume something that tastes sweet but doesn't contain any calories, your brain's pleasure pathway still gets activated by the sweet taste, but there's nothing to deactivate it because the calories never arrive.

Artificial sweeteners basically trick your body into thinking that it's going to receive sugar (calories). But when the sugar doesn't arrive, your body continues to signal that it needs more, which results in sugar cravings.

In 2004, a Purdue University study found that rats fed artificially sweetened liquids ate more high-calorie food than rats fed high-caloric sweetened liquids. The researchers believed the experience of drinking artificially sweetened liquids disrupted the animals' natural ability to compensate for the calories in the food.[10]

## The (Not-So) Skinny on Popular Artificial Sweeteners

• sucralose (Splenda)

A study published in the *Journal of Toxicology and Environmental Health* reported the devastating effects of the popular artificial sweetener sucralose. They found that rats fed dosages similar to the acceptable daily intake of Splenda approved by the FDA over a twelve-week period showed significantly lower levels of beneficial gut bacteria, compared to the control group.[11] Known as the *microbiome*, these beneficial bacteria that live in your gut serve to provide a host beneficial functions inside your body, including keeping your immune system functioning optimally.

• aspartame (AminoSweet)

Out of the thousands of food additives registered with the FDA, this artificial sweetener has received the majority of complaints. The most serious complaints relate to the neurological system because aspartame breaks down into free glutamate, an excitatory neurotransmitter in the brain. Constantly exciting your neurons will eventually lead them to become damaged or even killed.

- acesulfame potassium (Ace K)

This sweetener has gained in popularity in diet products, perhaps because it has undergone the least amount of scientific scrutiny. Often used in combination with other artificial sweeteners like aspartame, Ace K contains methylene chloride, a volatile organic compound known to cause nausea, mood problems, possibly some types of cancer, impaired liver and kidney function, problems with eyesight, and perhaps even autism.[12]

If that weren't enough, research in 2017 suggested that Ace K actually caused weight *gain* and affected the beneficial gut bacteria in mice.[13]

The takeaway: Ditch the "diet" products! Nothing created in a lab will ever be good for you. You can never fool Mother Nature.

*What about natural sweeteners like xylitol, erythritol, and stevia?*

Many health products contain xylitol and erythritol. These sugar alcohols have the ability to produce some undesirable side effects when ingested in large amounts, including digestive stress, headaches, and even weight gain. Erythritol can be produced from genetically modified corn. It's best to pass on these sweeteners.

My recommended (and safest) natural sweetener is stevia, a highly sweet herb derived from the leaf of the South American stevia plant. It's safe in its natural form and can be used to sweeten most dishes and drinks. Keep in mind that if you have insulin issues, high blood pressure, high cholesterol, or if you're overweight, you'd be better off avoiding all sweeteners, as any sweetener can decrease your sensitivity to insulin. Also, avoid stevia sweeteners that are cut with xylitol, dextrose, or even sugar.

Other natural sweeteners that can be good or bad include raw honey, dates, coconut sugar, and/or maple syrup; these are all-natural sweeteners. However, if you are trying to lose weight, have insulin issues, high blood pressure, and/or high cholesterol, it's best to avoid them altogether for now and consider adding them in extreme moderation down the road.

*What on earth should I be drinking?*

I may be stating the obvious, but you should be drinking water. How much water you should be drinking will depend on your activity level. As a general rule of thumb, try to drink at least a half ounce of water for every pound you weigh, as a starting point.

I'm often asked about coffee or tea. I think coffee and tea are great, as long as you don't add sugar. You can, however, add unsweetened coconut milk or virgin coconut oil to increase your healthier fats.

But remember that water should always be your main source of hydration, especially if your cortisol levels are out of control (more about that in chapter 12).

# CHAPTER 6

# The Skinny on Fat

There is a story told of a woman who brought home a leg of ham and was preparing it for Christmas dinner. She proceeded to cut it in half before placing it in the oven. Her husband, watching on, asked, "Why did you cut it in half? Is that so it cooks better in the middle?"

His wife paused a moment and then answered, "I don't really know. That's just what I've always done. I saw my mother doing that when I was a girl."

Later, her parents arrived for Christmas dinner, and she raised the question, "Mom, why did you cut the leg of ham in half before placing it in the oven?"

"I don't really know," her mother replied. "Your grandma used to do that, so it's just something I've always done. There must be a reason for it."

Later, the family all traveled to Grandma's house to share Christmas dessert. During a lull in the conversation, the wife asked her grandmother, "Grandma, why did you teach Mom to cut the leg of ham in half before cooking it?"

"Well," replied the grandmother, "when your mother was a girl, my oven was very small, and I couldn't fit the whole leg in without cutting it in half."

I like to tell this story because I see a parallel between it and a number of assumptions we hold on to regarding health, fitness, and nutrition, despite evidence that doesn't support them.

You may hold a lot of false assumptions when it comes to fat. You may believe that fat will make you gain weight or that it will "clog" your arteries and cause a heart attack or stroke. That isn't true!

## The Low-Fat Craze

In the 1950s, higher rates of death from coronary heart disease in American men led to studies of the role of dietary factors, including cholesterol, calories, fats, carbohydrates, vitamins, and minerals in influencing coronary heart disease. By the 1960s, two theories were being championed as potential causes. One theory was that sugars were the primary cause, and the other was that it was dietary fat and cholesterol. But by 1980, the first *Dietary Guidelines for Americans* was published, focusing on reducing total fat, saturated fat, and dietary cholesterol for the prevention of coronary heart disease. And it appears that the theory on sugars contributing to coronary heart disease was buried by some very powerful influences, namely the sugar industry.[14]

The result was that following a low-fat, higher-sugar diet caused heart disease to skyrocket to even greater levels. Maybe it wasn't the fat after all. Maybe it was all the sugars and grains we added to our diets. It's time to start looking at fat from a different perspective.

*Fat is great on one condition—that it comes from a healthy source!*

Fat is essential not only to our bodies' ability to function normally internally but also at the deeper level of the cell. Healthy sources of fat help your brain and your gastrointestinal system, and they help you build your hormones and are anti-inflammatory. They are also the preferred source of fuel for your brain. In fact, every cell in your body—approximately 70 trillion—has a cell membrane made of fat that allows nutrients to go into the cell and waste to exit.

## Bad Fats to Avoid: Any Fat That Has Been Altered

- hydrogenated and partially hydrogenated oils

Also known as trans-fats, hydrogenated or partially hydrogenated oils are synthetic fatty acids that have been chemically altered to prevent melting at room temperature and to give foods a longer shelf life. They aren't naturally occurring fats, and you'll find them in a lot of packaged foods that contain fat. Trans-fats prevent the synthesis of prostacyclin, which is necessary to keep your blood flowing through your arteries. When your arteries cannot produce prostacyclin, blood clots form, and you may succumb to sudden death. That sure sounds like a heart attack to me.

Mounting research suggests there is *no* safe limit for trans fats. This makes it an even greater concern than sugar, which your body can safely handle in small doses. Trans fats can also increase insulin resistance.[15]

*But the label says "No Trans Fats"!*

*Great*: In 2006, food manufacturers were forced to list the amount of trans-fats in their product.

*Not So Great*: Food manufacturers manipulated the law to allow labels to read "trans-fat free" if a product contained less than 500 milligrams of trans-fats per serving.

*The Scam:* Food manufacturers decreased product serving size to make the trans-fats disappear from the label.

*The Takeaway*: Always look at the ingredients on the back label, and never fall for the slick advertising on the front!

- rancid vegetable oils

These oils are listed on the label as corn oil, soybean oil, sunflower oil, peanut oil, canola oil, or simply vegetable oil. The problem with these fats is that when they are heated at high temperatures, such as frying, they become unstable and inflammatory, and they will cause the oxidation of cholesterol inside the body. Cholesterol isn't destructive until it becomes oxidized, but even when these oils aren't oxidized by frying, they can oxidize inside the body.

- fats from grain-fed beef

People often say, "You are what you eat." However, when it comes to the fats that come from meat, it should be stated that you are what *they* ate.

Think about it: If you want to make a person gain weight, give him a diet high in sugars and grains. If you want to pack the pounds on a cow, give a cow a diet high in grains too.

Not only are commercially raised cattle fed grains in the form of corn and soy, but cattle also can be given hormones to help pack on the pounds in a short amount of time, as well as antibiotics to help them survive their unsanitary living conditions. All of this can end up in the meat you eat.

One of the other major differences between grain-fed beef and grass-fed beef is the type of fat present in the beef. Grass-fed beef will have a significantly higher (and healthier) ratio of omega-3 fatty acids than grain-fed beef (more about that later).

In addition, grass-fed beef will contain higher amounts of vitamins and minerals such as vitamin A, vitamin E, potassium, zinc, iron, phosphorus, and sodium.

The bottom line: Grain-fed beef will promote more inflammation and generally be more toxic. It's much more important to go organic when it comes to beef and get healthier sources of fat than to go organic on your fruits and vegetables.

## Good Fats to Add: Fats That Have Never Been Altered

- extra-virgin olive oil

Extra-virgin olive oil is a smart fat to include in your diet in a nonheated form, such as in a salad dressing. *Extra virgin* means the oil has undergone extraction by pressing, not heating. However, if you heat virgin olive oil to over 250 degrees, you run the risk of creating oxidized oil that can do your body more harm than good by creating inflammation. It's better to use this type of oil to add finishing touches to food rather than heating it at high temperatures.

- virgin coconut oil and MCT oil (remember this one for later)

Don't be scared away by the fact that coconut and MCT (medium-chain triglycerides) oils are primarily composed of saturated fat. There's a difference between an altered saturated fat, like the fat in hydrogenated oils, and the saturated fat found in coconut oil. In fact, there is no evidence that naturally occurring saturated fats like coconut oil have any negative impact on your health. On the contrary, evidence abounds that it is actually healthy for you.

### The Amazing Benefits of Coconut Oil

- promotes heart health
- promotes weight loss
- supports your immune system with its antiviral, antibacterial, and antiprotozoal properties
- supports a healthy metabolism
- provides your body with an immediate energy source that is not stored as fat
- keeps your skin healthy and youthful-looking when applied to the skin
- supports the proper function of your thyroid gland (a big problem today)

Coconut oil and high-quality MCT oil are stable at high temperatures and can be used for frying, making them the go-to oils when cooking. When in doubt about which one to cook with, coconut oil—in solid form at room temperature—always is the right choice.

- cold-compressed and expeller-pressed oils

These oils have been extracted by pressing, not heating. Look for these in healthier versions of packaged foods, but always read the label. There may be a lot of sugar in them, even if they are organic. In addition, avoid heating them at high temperatures. Some good ones to look for are pumpkin, sesame seed, avocado, hemp seed, and flaxseed oils.

- raw nuts and seeds

Nuts and seeds are extremely healthy, and most people don't eat enough of them. They are a great natural source of vitamins, minerals, protein, and fiber and are packed with healthy fats. A word of caution, however: Make sure the nuts and seeds you consume are raw, not roasted. To maximize the nutrients you get from nuts and seeds, soak them in distilled or purified water overnight. This helps neutralize enzyme inhibitors that may affect digestion and absorption of the nutrients. It also can help reduce the amount of pesticides on them if they are not organically grown.

Here are some great nuts to consume:

| Tree Nut (grams per ounce) | Fat | Protein | Carbs |
|---|---|---|---|
| macadamias | 22 | 2 | 4 |
| pecans | 20 | 3 | 4 |
| pine nuts | 20 | 4 | 4 |

| brazil nuts | 19 | 4 | 3 |
|---|---|---|---|
| walnuts | 18 | 4 | 4 |
| hazelnuts | 17 | 3 | 5 |
| cashews | 13 | 4 | 9 |
| almonds | 14 | 6 | 6 |
| pistachios | 13 | 6 | 8 |

Some of the healthiest seeds include the following:
- flax
- chia
- hemp
- sunflower
- pumpkin
- sesame

Do "nut" eat peanuts (terrible pun intended). Peanuts actually are legumes, not a nut. Peanuts can contain a carcinogenic mold called *aflatoxin*, and they are notorious for being one of the most pesticide-contaminated crops. If you eat peanuts, organic roasted peanuts or peanut butter is your safest bet.

I prefer to eat organic nut butters, such as almond butter, sunflower-seed butter, and walnut butter.

- grass-fed beef (and full-fat dairy), cage-free chicken (and eggs), pacific or wild-caught fish

The fats and proteins from these sources are less toxic, and these sources have a major difference in the essential fatty-acid makeup.

Essential fatty acids are fats that your body cannot manufacture, so they must come from dietary sources. Grass-fed and cage-free sources will have higher ratios of omega-3 fatty acids, as compared to omega-6 fatty acids. Research has shown that the farther people's essential fatty-acids ratio is from 4:1 (omega-6 to omega-3), the more general health problems they have. Grass-fed beef, for example, has a ratio of 3:1 while grain-feed beef has a ratio of up to 20:1.

In short, naturally sourced fats are rich in all the fats now proven to be health-enhancing and low in the fats that have been linked with disease.

## Farm-Raised vs. Wild-Caught Fish

| Farm-Raised vs. Wild-Caught | Farm-Raised | Wild-Caught |
|---|---|---|
| Nutrition | Lower levels of protein, omega-3s and found to contain more fats | Higher levels of omega 3s and less fats |
| Feed | Fed fishmeal derived from conventionally grown crops most likely containing pesticides, herbicides, and GMOs | Find natural food found in the wild |
| PCBs | These highly toxic compounds are eight times more present in farm-raised fish | Contain very low levels of PCBs |
| Mercury | Lower levels of mercury usually are found in farm fish | Some fish, especially salmon, may contain mercury; recommended to not eat fish every day |

## Get Your Essential Fatty Acids in Balance

EPA and DHA are two of the most critical essential fatty acids to consume. These omega-3 essential fatty acids have tremendous health benefits, including the following:

- They help to improve inflammation, pain, kidney function, MS, RA, psoriasis, heart disease, asthma, diabetes, allergies, arthritis, immune system, gene expression, sleep, and memory, among other benefits.[16]
- They help improve symptoms of bipolar disorder and depression by blocking the abnormal signaling in the brain that is present in depression and mania. Essential fatty acids also help to boost serotonin levels in the brain.[17]
- They help to reduce the risk of Alzheimer's disease and dementia by protecting the vascular system, reducing brain inflammation, and aiding in the regeneration of nerve cells.[18]
- They help reduce risk of sudden cardiac death by up to 90 percent.[19]

How much should you take?

If you are eating two servings of wild- or Pacific-caught fish per week, you are most likely getting enough in your diet. If you're like me and don't like eating fish, consider supplementing with a pharmaceutical-grade omega supplement, with the goal of getting around 1–2 grams of EPA and DHA per day.

For more information on the omega-3 fatty acid supplements I recommend and where to shop for healthy fats, visit the resource page at *Transformation28.net*.

## Avocados 101: Superfood or "Superfad"?

The avocado is a fruit that's exceptionally high in fat, but don't let that fool you. The avocado is low in sugar and high in fiber, so it won't spike your blood sugar. Rich in monosaturated fat (like olive oil), the primary fat is oleic acid, which helps fight inflammation and protect against heart disease, type 2 diabetes, cancer, and arthritis.

Avocados also are high in vitamins and minerals, as well as carotenoids, which help with overall eye health.

*The bottom line:* Avocados are definitely a superfood to help target inflammation and are a great addition to your diet to help with weight loss, making it a great food to incorporate in your nutrition plan.

*A word of caution*: Avocados do contain FODMAPs (fermentable oligo, di-, monosaccharides and polyols), which are a type of carbohydrate that certain people find difficult to digest. If you notice any cramping or bloating after consuming avocados, it might be a good idea to avoid them altogether.

# CHAPTER 7

# You Need Protein (but Not Too Much)

Proteins are the building blocks for the muscles, organs, and cells inside your body. If you don't consume enough protein, you'll suffer from muscle wasting, you'll have a weakened immune system, and you'll have brittle hair, nails, and skin.

You can consume too much protein, which will turn to sugar and keep your insulin levels high.

How much protein should you be getting per day?

Try to limit your daily intake to between .5 and .75 grams of protein per pound of lean body mass (your total weight minus your fat weight) per day. For the elderly and those participating in a regular exercise program, I recommend increasing your protein intake to .75–1.0 grams of protein per pound of lean body mass per day.

For example, a person doing strenuous exercise four to five times per week with 100 pounds of lean body mass would need between 75 and 100 grams of protein per day (more on how to calculate this in chapter 8).

The best types of protein will come from the best sources of fat—that's more natural sources like grass-fed beef and dairy, cage-free chicken and eggs, Pacific- or wild-caught fish, wild game, organic turkey, and grass-fed whey protein.

For vegans, beans and lentils (in moderation), raw nuts and seeds, a vegan plant protein supplement (rice, pea, and/or hemp), and fermented soy products will help you fulfill your protein needs.

## M-m-m-m … Bacon—and Other Toxic Proteins to Avoid

I'll admit that bacon tastes amazing, but it's best to avoid bacon and other pork products, processed meats, and shellfish. These foods are almost always high in toxicity and/or nitrites, a potentially cancer-causing substance.

What about soy?

Once touted as a health food, the use of soy has been called into question over the years. Consider some of the evidence:

- Soy is high in phytic acid and trypsin inhibitors, leading to digestive issues such as diarrhea, gas, and bloating; it also may block the absorption of minerals.
- Soy is a phytoestrogen, which can increase the estrogen levels in your body (not only for women but also for men and children). In today's toxic world, I've found very few people who suffer with low estrogen but many who suffer with too much.
- Soy has been associated with thyroid problems, leading to the formation of an enlarged thyroid (goiter). If you have a thyroid issue, avoid this food.
- Most soy products in the United States are genetically modified and will therefore contain more glyphosate, a potentially cancer-causing chemical.

## An Easy Way to Get Quality Protein: Whey

One of the easiest ways to fulfill your daily protein requirements is by consuming whey protein. Derived from milk, whey protein has been found to be one of the greatest, most bioavailable forms of protein today. Whey protein is believed to help increase energy expenditure, suppress appetite, aid in detoxification, and help promote weight loss. Whey protein is rich in the amino acid leucine, a great protein for increasing muscle mass.

As with any other animal product, however, where the protein comes from and how the animal was raised plays a huge role in whether it will be good for you. As with your fats, whey protein should come from grass-fed, organic sources.

I've used a high-quality whey protein with my patients for years, and the results are astounding. They find it easy to use as a meal replacement, and it removes the worry about food preparation while they are detoxing off sugars and grains. It's one of the reasons I routinely see people lose up to twenty pounds in just twenty-eight days and improve their health biomarkers in just a few weeks.

One thing is certain: If you can make healthy eating easier, you're much more likely to change for good!

For those looking for a vegan alternative to whey, I recommend pea, hemp, or brown rice protein.

For more information on which whey and vegan protein I personally use and recommend, visit the resource page at *Transformation28.net.*

# CHAPTER 8

# Putting a Plan in Place with Your Nutrition

Now that you understand the good and bad about your macronutrients (carbohydrates, fats, and proteins), the next step is to figure out the ratio of these macronutrients you should be consuming.

Here is where I recommend starting for anyone looking to improve their nutrition:

- 25 percent of your total calories from carbohydrates
- 50 percent of your total calories from fat
- 25 percent of your total calories from protein

You may find other available plans even more beneficial than the one described above. Some people may find the Zone diet (40 percent carbohydrates, 30 percent fat, 30 percent protein) or the ketogenic diet (5 percent carbohydrates, 70 percent fat, 25 percent protein) extremely helpful. This will depend on certain health conditions, your exercise volume, and/or your preferred type of exercise. You always can modify your macronutrient breakdown later on. After all, you have the rest of your life to see what your body prefers, based on where you are with your health.

One thing, however, should never change, and that's the quality of food you should be eating!

## Finding Your Target Macronutrient Ratios and Daily Caloric Intake

When finding your target macronutrient ratios, you first need to understand how many calories are in a gram of carbohydrates, fat, and protein:

- carbs = 4 calories per gram
- protein = 4 calories per gram
- fat = 9 calories per gram

1) Calculate how much protein you need per day based on your lean body mass. To find your lean body mass, first measure your body weight and body fat percentage. Use the following simple calculation to measure your lean body mass:

- body weight x body fat % = fat mass
- body weight – fat mass = lean body mass
- lean body mass x (.5–1.0) = grams of protein needed per day

If you're unsure how much protein you need per day, reread chapter 7 to find your specific protein needs.

2) Calculate how many carbohydrates you need per day. Since it's recommended that your carbohydrate and protein intake each equal 25 percent of your daily caloric intake, and carbohydrates and protein both contain equal calories per gram, your recommended carbohydrates will equal your protein needed per day. (Pretty easy!)

3) Calculate how much fat you need per day. This can get tricky, but here's a simple formula:

- Add your recommended grams of protein and carbohydrates and multiply by 4 calories, which equals 50 percent of your total calories
- Since fat will equal the other 50 percent of your total calories, divide that number by 9 calories/gram equaling your total fat grams per day.

Let's look at an example:

A two-hundred-pound male has a body fat percentage of 25 percent. He gets high-intensity exercise four to five times per week and needs .75 grams of protein per pound of lean body mass per day.

- 200 x .25 = 50 pounds of fat mass
- 200 pounds – 50 pounds = 150 pounds lean body mass
- 150 pounds x .75 g/protein per pound of lean body mass = 112.5 grams of protein per day
- grams of carbohydrates per day = 112.5 g
- grams of carbohydrates + grams of protein = 225 grams of carbohydrate and protein per day
- 225 grams x 4 calories per gram = 900 calories of carbohydrates and protein per day (50 percent of total calories)
- total fat calories per day = 900 calories (50 percent of total calories)
- 900 calories/9 calories per gram = 100 grams of fat per day

*Total Recommended Macros*
112.5 grams of protein per day
112.5 grams of carbohydrates per day
100 grams of fat per day

Total calories per day = 1800

*What's the best way to measure body fat percentage?*

There are numerous techniques to measure body fat percentage, and each technique has its benefits and drawbacks. I personally recommend bioelectrical impedance analysis (or BIA) for its accuracy and ease of use. The most accurate BIAs will involve the full body, specifically the InBody analyzer, but you can use a more inexpensive handheld unit called the Omron Body Fat Analyzer. While not as accurate as the InBody, it will give you a fairly good idea of your overall body fat percentage if you use it for both pre- and post-analysis.

## A Quick Note

You may be asking, "Is that all I get to eat?" The answer is yes. Once you start to reduce your sugar and grain intake, you find yourself less hungry and desiring less food that ever before. Give it four weeks. After that, you can add in more nutrients. Just make sure to keep the ratios balanced.

## Hormone-Based Nutrition Recap

Eat meat and vegetables, nuts and seeds, some fruit, little starch, and no sugar.

Keep your intake to levels that support exercise but not body fat.

Now it makes sense, doesn't it? I'll give you the plan at the end of the book to be successful for twenty-eight days.

For a simple online calculator to determine your recommended macronutrients, visit the resource page at *Transformation 28.net.*

# CHAPTER 9

# Your "Big Why"

Let's take a step back. You might be thinking that this seems too hard.

I've helped thousands of people who thought it was too hard; it was hard for me too. The reason it was hard was because my *why* wasn't big enough. For many years I tried to diet and exercise for the sole purpose of looking good in a Speedo. (FYI, no one looks good in a Speedo.) That wasn't a very good why.

It's been said that you can accomplish the how when your why is big enough. I fully agree.

Have you ever seen people make amazing life transformations? They go from being one hundred pounds overweight and lying on the couch to losing one hundred pounds and running 5Ks and obstacle courses.

The conversation always comes around to the question "Why did you do it?"

You never hear them say "I wanted to look better" or "I wanted to feel better" or "I wanted to fit into my clothes again." Rather, their reason generally sounds like this: "I wasn't going to be there for my daughter's wedding" or "I couldn't play with my kids anymore."

They had a reason that was bigger than themselves. That's called your *big why*.

A patient once came to see me who was suffering from advanced lung cancer; she had the goal of getting healthier. She reeked of smoke, and I could see her cigarette lighter and cigarettes in her purse. When I told her the first thing she needed to do was quit smoking, she said she couldn't because it was too hard. I asked her, "Could you do it if someone threatened to kill you if you took one drag from that cigarette in your purse?"

Without giving it a second thought, she said, "Of course I could because my life would depend on it." And that's when the light bulb went on.

Health is rarely achieved in one monumental decision but rather the small decisions we make daily to choose a better life and better health. Once you see that your bad decisions are nothing more than a slow form of suicide, you'll see that your excuses are just rationalizations that keep you sick and keep you from realizing what's possible with better health.

Being healthier, or wanting more energy, or even wanting to lose some weight is not a big enough why. Rather, what would you be able to *accomplish* if you were healthier or had more energy?

What is your big why? Write it down. Seriously. Write it down. Before you move on, you need to know exactly what it is so that you can anchor your mind when the going gets tough—and it will get tough when you decide to take the T28 Challenge at the end of the book.

# CHAPTER 10

# Exercise: You Know You Need It, but Why Don't You Do It?

Let's say scientists could create a new breakthrough treatment that did the following:

- reduced blood pressure
- reduced cholesterol and triglycerides
- reduced fat
- improved blood sugar and insulin sensitivity
- increased bone mass
- improved energy, sleep, and mood
- improved chronic pain
- made you smarter

Would you want this breakthrough treatment? Of course you would!

Well, this breakthrough treatment is available right now without a prescription. It's called *exercise*.

It doesn't take a scientist to realize the amazing benefits that exercise has to offer. In fact, exercise improves all areas of health, both physically and mentally. Exercise outperforms just about every drug on the market today, including drugs for depression.[20]

When was the last time your doctor prescribed exercise instead of a pill for what was ailing you? He or she might have offered you a tepid suggestion, but chances are your doctor has not given you a detailed prescription on how to get into the best shape of your life in just a few short weeks.

Most people are painfully aware they should exercise, so why don't they? Take a look at the most common exercise myths and the real truth. Chances are you've believed all of these myths at some point in your life.

## Exercise Myths and Truths

*Myth No. 1*: Exercise hurts.

*Truth*: Exercise reduces pain and improves arthritis.

When people tell me that they don't exercise because it hurts, I always wonder what the word *hurt* means to them, exactly. Do they mean it makes them uncomfortable? Sometimes it's necessary to get uncomfortable to broaden your horizons. After all, the science is clear: The more you depart from a state of resting homeostasis, the greater the results you'll get from an exercise session. This is not to say that if you've never exercised or haven't exercised in a long time you should do an extremely intense workout. Many people have to spend several weeks getting into shape just to begin the process. Sometimes it's best to take it slow. After all, Rome (or arthritis) wasn't built in a day.

Furthermore, it is important to know your limitations and to stay in tune with your body. If you have a severely degenerated knee, then performing full-depth squats or box jumps won't be your cup of tea. However, you can safely scale any movement to help your body acclimate. It's critical that a degenerated joint be exposed to constant motion. If you don't use it, you lose it. When done correctly, exercise actually alleviates pain and arthritis.

How many times have you said, "I can't do [name your form of exercise] because I have a bad [name your arthritic body part]"?

One of the worst things you can do for an arthritic joint is to stop moving it. If you've ever broken a bone and had it casted and immobilized for even a few weeks, you probably noticed that the joints and muscles around it became stiff, painful, and weak. Doesn't that sound like arthritis? The answer to healing a joint is to move it. After all, motion is life to the body.

*Myth No. 2*: I don't have time to exercise.
*Truth*: Achieving incredible fitness levels takes only a few minutes a day.

Research shows that to get the best results from an exercise program with the goal of achieving incredible fitness, the way to go is to perform high-intensity, short-duration functional exercise. In as little as three to fifteen minutes a day, you can have a profound impact on your fitness levels. You get a big return on your investment in the shortest amount of time.

But to get these results, it won't be an easy couple of minutes.

*Myth No. 3*: I can't afford a gym membership.
*Truth*: You can get an incredible workout with little to no exercise equipment.

You don't need a gym to achieve a higher level of fitness and health, and I say that as a gym owner. While I'm a huge fan of going to the gym for the accountability and coaching, at the end of the day, exercise is free. It doesn't have to cost you a penny. You can do workouts at home, at a park, or on the road with little to no equipment (just watch out for cars!). The opportunities are endless.

# CHAPTER 11

# What Is Fitness, Anyway?

Ask one hundred people what they believe fitness is, and you'll probably get a hundred different answers. Some will say it's the ability to run a 5K. Others might say it's the ability to pick up a heavy weight off the floor. Still others might suggest it's having the ability to energetically dance to bad '80s music while wearing tights (hopefully a very small minority). Regardless of people's answers, not a lot of people can clearly define it.

Up until the last decade, fitness never was clearly defined, and it's impossible to work toward the goal of fitness if we don't know what it is.

Here's what I believe is *the best* definition of fitness:

*It's the ability to do work across broad time and movement domains.*

Work is defined by the ability to apply a force on an object for a specific distance. The force might be your own body weight, a barbell, a kettlebell, a dumbbell, or maybe even a wheelbarrow. Multiply that force by the distance traveled, and now you have work. Your ability to perform this work in the shortest amount of time possible (intensity) and utilizing a number of different movements is what fitness truly is.

While the number of possible movements to incorporate into your fitness routine is infinite, it might include the following:

- monostructural movements: running, swimming, jumping rope, rowing, or biking
- weight lifting movements: squatting, Olympic lifting, kettlebells, or dumbbells

- gymnastic movements: pull-ups, push-ups, sit-ups, handstands

Well-rounded fitness should not only give you better cardiovascular endurance, but it should also help to improve stamina, strength, flexibility, power, speed, coordination, agility, balance, and accuracy.

And as a result of well-rounded fitness, you should be able to achieve better hormone function, stronger muscles, more muscle mass, less fat, improved sleep and energy, better mobility, and a stronger mental framework (arguably, the most important).

## The Best (and Worst) Way to Exercise to Achieve Fitness

The first thing people think when they have the desire to get into better shape is that they have to spend hours and hours in the fat-burning zone on the treadmill (or "dreadmill," as I call it), elliptical, or stair-climber in order to lose weight. We call that steady-state exercise. While doing this form of exercise has its benefits, there are some major drawbacks.

Perhaps the biggest drawback when doing steady-state exercise is that it raises a stress hormone called cortisol (remember this hormone). While it's a great hormone in an acute crisis, chronically elevated cortisol can have devastating effects on the body over time. Chronically elevated cortisol will stimulate your appetite, cause muscle wasting, increase fat storage, diminish the immune system, and decrease testosterone and human growth hormone (hormones responsible for fat burning and muscle building).

Even with all the negatives already mentioned, one additional drawback perks up a lot of people's ears: Chronically elevated cortisol *causes* the deposition of cellulite.[21]

The big question, then, becomes this: How can we get all the amazing benefits of exercise without any of the drawbacks?

The answer is high-intensity, short-duration, functional exercise.

**The Case for High-Intensity, Short-Duration, Functional Exercise for Fat Loss**

While most people consider how many calories they burn as the benchmark for effective exercise and fat loss, it's simply not the case. What matters most is the muscle-building and fat-burning hormone response *after* you exercise. Known as human growth hormone, this hormone is influenced by the intensity with which you exercise. With steady-state exercise, you'll be in the fat-burning zone for minutes. With high-intensity, short-duration, functional exercise, you'll train your body to be in the fat-burning zone for hours after you're done with your workout.

Research over the last twenty years is finally uncovering what's been true since the dawn of man: In the realm of fitness, high intensity is best.

- High-intensity exercise achieved superior fat loss, compared to moderate steady-state exercise. [22]
- There is a greater increase in fat expenditure after high-intensity exercise due to the release of human growth hormone. [23]
- There was a significant loss in body fat in a group that exercised at a high intensity of 80–90 percent of maximal heart rate, while no significant change in body fat was found in the lower-intensity group that exercised at 60–70 percent of maximal heart rate, despite performing the same amount of work. [24]
- High-intensity exercise is superior for reversing the symptoms of metabolic syndrome, also known as prediabetes. [25]

*The bottom line*: When it comes to exercise, what matters most is the amount of work you perform in the shortest amount of time. This equals intensity, and intensity equals results!

**Functional Exercise: Exercise That Makes You Better at Life**

Exercise should not only be about fat loss. Exercise should help you become better at everyday life. If you took an inventory of the activities of your day, you'd notice that you need to perform a multitude of movements well. You need to be able to get up off of a chair, pick up groceries, play with your kids or grandkids, push a lawnmower, bend over in a garden, or swing a golf club.

The following are some movements that you need to be able to do to stay functional and move well throughout your entire life, not only to avoid the nursing home but to excel at life in general:

- squats and all their variations
- lunges
- dead lifts
- overhead presses
- kettlebell swings
- burpees
- push-ups
- pull-ups and rope climbs
- jumping activities, like jumping rope or box jumps
- running, swimming, and rowing
- core work: sit-ups, planks, and arch holds

While not an exhaustive list, if you practiced and mastered just these movements, then mixed these elements three to six times per week in as many combinations as your creativity will allow, and then combined them into a short, intense workout lasting anywhere from three to fifteen minutes, you'd be well on your way to achieving the absolute best fitness of your life.

## What's the Best Time to Exercise and What Should I Eat Afterward?

Your first priority should be to exercise whenever you can get it done. From a fat-loss perspective, however, the best time to exercise is in the morning on an empty stomach. You will be in a fasting state; your human growth hormone will be at its highest, and your insulin level will be at its lowest. This will make you primed and ready for fat burning and muscle building immediately after you are done working out.

At the conclusion of your workout, you'll want to keep your human growth hormone as high as possible for as long as possible, if fat loss is your goal. One way to stop the fat-burning process is to consume sugars and grains immediately after exercise. Therefore, avoid any sugar, grains, and fruit for at least two hours in order to let your hormones continue to work for you and not against you. I often consume whey protein and healthy fats to give my body the building blocks to repair and recover.

## You're Never "Too Far Gone"

You may be thinking that you're too far gone or that you are too old. Don't let that become your excuse. Maybe the following story will inspire you and give you hope. I know it's an inspiration for me. Let me introduce to you Rex and Mary Pat.

Rex and Mary Pat started their journey toward achieving amazing health and fitness with all kinds of health problems. Rex was on medications for asthma and acid reflux and was well on his way to becoming a type 2 diabetic. Mary Pat had watched her two siblings pass away from lifestyle-induced disease. At one point, her knees were so arthritic that she needed the help of a walker to move around.

After applying the principles outlined in this book, Rex and Mary Pat lost over 150 pounds, combined. Not only that, but Rex was able to climb a fifteen-foot rope with ease, and Mary Pat was able to run a 5K in under forty minutes!

Did I mention they are older than sixty years of age?

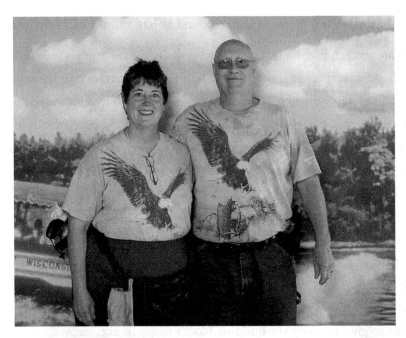

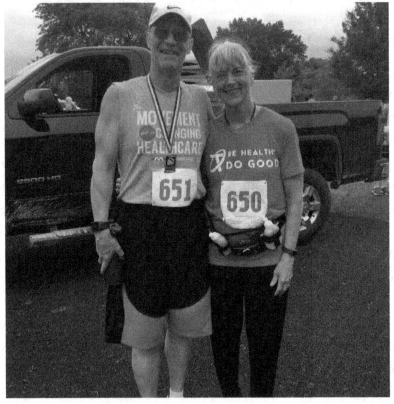

# CHAPTER 12

# Stress, Cortisol, and Vitamin D

## Get Your Stress under Control

Stress is a killer, and the hormone known as cortisol can get out of control during times of stress, including when you do long-duration, steady-state exercise. Produced by the adrenal glands, cortisol's functions include blood pressure regulation, proper metabolism of glucose, maintenance of blood sugar, maintenance of the immune system, and more. Usually, you have high amounts of cortisol in your body in the morning, and it decreases as night approaches. Cortisol is one of the hormones released in your body during stressful events, and some of the positive effects of this include a higher pain threshold, a rush of energy, increased immunity, and an improved memory. While this is a great response when a bear is chasing you, it's not so great when the bear chases you for months on end. While I don't know any circumstance where a bear might chase you for months, I do know a lot of circumstances that produce a similar stress response—like a lack of sleep, relationship stress, job stress, too much exercise, and too much caffeine every day.

Cortisol will make you fat and hungry. When your body constantly produces an abnormally high amount of cortisol, your normal cortisol production can be disrupted. Instead of having more cortisol in the morning and less cortisol in the evening, the pattern of cortisol in your body can be altered. Since this hormone is responsible for providing you with energy, it also stimulates the metabolism of carbohydrates and fats.

Cortisol also helps your body release insulin. These internal activities can lead to an appetite increase, so the longer cortisol is at work in your body, the more hunger pangs you likely will feel.

Cortisol also increases blood sugar when you're feeling stressed. When the stressful event is over and your blood sugar level is still high, the excess glucose gets stored as fat. Some studies have shown that excess cortisol not only leads to fat deposition, but the hormone also can affect where the fat is stored. Researchers believe that individuals who gain weight due to cortisol are more likely to have abdominal fat.

## Getting Your Cortisol Under Control

Here are five ways to get your cortisol under control:

1. Sleep: Get at least seven to nine hours of sleep each night in compete darkness. Avoid any artificial white light while you sleep.
2. Reduce stress: Whether a bear is chasing you in the forest or you're experiencing stress at work, your brain perceives *any* stress as a threat to your life. Stress is not the event; it's how you choose to respond to it.
3. Avoid long-duration workouts: Workouts lasting more than forty-five to sixty minutes will increase cortisol and lead to adrenal fatigue over time. Keep your workouts short and intense, and schedule at least one to two rest days per week.
4. Kick the caffeine: Caffeine consumption can elevate cortisol levels. Quitting caffeine cold turkey can cause some intense side effects, such as headaches, nausea, anxiety, and sleepiness. If the cold-turkey method doesn't sound very enticing, try reducing your caffeine intake by 25 percent every two days in order to decrease withdrawal effects.
5. Take supplements that support the adrenal glands and lower cortisol.

The following supplements help lower cortisol and improve adrenal function:

- Omega-3 fatty acids: Omega-3 fatty acids have countless benefits, and lowering cortisol is one of them. I recommend getting at least 1–2 grams of omega-3 fatty acids of EPA and DHA per day; and in cases of elevated inflammation, 2–3 grams per day.

- B vitamins: A quality methylated B vitamin has been known to support healthy adrenal function, while also fighting against high cortisol levels. B vitamins also have been known to promote a sense of calm while naturally boosting energy, making this group of vitamins essential to those dealing with high levels of stress.

- Ashwagandha: Animal and human studies have demonstrated that ashwagandha has anti-inflammatory, antioxidant, adaptogenic (cortisol-reducing), antipyretic (fever-reducing), and antimicrobial (germ-fighting) benefits, as well as its antianxiety and mood-elevating capabilities.[26]

- GABA: Short for gamma amino butyric acid, this neurotransmitter has a calming effect on the central nervous system and is useful for those who have issues "turning off" their brains before sleep.

- L-Phenylalanine and Tyrosine: These amino acids support the production of dopamine, norepinephrine, and epinephrine. Increased dopamine is thought to improve concentration, movement, emotional response, attention, and focus. Dopamine is the source of the brain's power and energy and is useful for people who typically wake up feeling tired in the morning.

## Vitamin D: The Vitamin You're Probably Deficient In

As if there's not enough research out there about the benefits of vitamin D and the role it plays in increasing the effectiveness of the immune system, helping the body fight cancer cell formation, and preventing autoimmunity, there's more.

Research now suggests that the higher a person's vitamin D levels, the higher the levels of adiponectin, a hormone that regulates fat burning.[27]

Could the reason that you can't lose weight and shed fat be because you lack sufficient vitamin D?

The best way to discover how much vitamin D you should be taking is by measuring the levels of vitamin D in your blood, which ideally should be between 60 and 70 ng/dl. Typically, I recommend at least 5,000 IU per day, with probiotics to help with absorption, in order to achieve optimal levels.

For more information on which supplements I use personally use and recommend for overcoming stress and optimal vitamin D levels visit the resource page at *Transformation28.net*.

# CHAPTER 13

# The T28 Challenge: Transformation in Twenty-Eight Days

Now it's time to get to work and put your newfound knowledge into action. After all, knowledge is nothing without action.

The goal of the T28 Challenge is simple: to help you become an efficient fat-burner, to reduce or eliminate your sugar cravings, to help you finally begin to lose fat, and to turn health-damaging habits into health-building habits. It takes at least twenty-eight days to build new habits, and that's why it's called the T28 Challenge.

*A word of caution:* The T28 Challenge is *not* designed to do the following:

- solve all your health issues (although many of them will improve)
- be a diet plan for the rest of your life
- turn you into a culinary wizard
- bring world peace (although I do believe it will lead many people to becoming healthier and happier)

With the simple goals of the T28 Challenge, I want to make it easier, not harder, for you to follow through. Over the next twenty-eight days, you'll notice a lot of changes, and you'll experience some withdrawal symptoms. That's why making it simple and easy to follow through with the T28 Challenge plan is the best way to tackle your health issues.

*Beware*: The T28 Challenge plan is *not* for those who want to try it out or see how it goes. If that's you, I can tell you that you will fail. You will need to be all in.

Are you *all in*?

Have you written down your big why?

Are you really ready?

Then let's do this!

# CHAPTER 14

# The Twenty-Eight-Day
# Nutrition and Fitness Plan

First, you'll need to go back to chapter 8 and calculate your daily protein, fat, and carbohydrate requirements for the day. For an online macronutrient calculator, visit the resources page of *Transformation28.net*.

Current weight _____ pounds

Current body fat: _____ percent

Total lean mass: _____ pounds

My recommended total protein: _____ grams

My recommended total carbs: _____ grams

My recommended total fat: _____ grams

My recommended total calories: _____

**Breakfast and Lunch**

Consume one T28 smoothie.

- 1 scoop (women)/1.5 scoops (men) of grass-fed whey protein or vegan protein
- 1/2 scoop of evaporated greens (to help with inflammation)
- 1 tablespoon of MCT oil (remember this one?)
- 8 ounces (women)/12 ounces (men) of unsweetened coconut milk (available at any grocery store)

Combine the ingredients into a blender bottle (the coconut milk first), mix, and enjoy!

## Snacks (choose two of the following per day)

- 1/4 cup (women)/1/3 cup (men) of raw nuts (approximately a handful)
- 1/2 cup of any type of berries
- 1 medium-size Granny Smith apple or grapefruit

*Caution:* If you are currently taking a cholesterol-lowering drug, avoid grapefruit altogether, as it can increase the drug's side effects.

## Dinner

- fish, chicken, beef, turkey, or eggs (grass-fed, pastured, free-range, or cage-free is best)
- vegetables—as many as you want until you feel full (raw, steamed, or sautéed in coconut oil)
- if you need to increase your fat, add another tablespoon of coconut oil or MCT oil, or enjoy an avocado

## How Much Protein at Dinner?

Men: Daily recommended protein minus the 60 grams (from the smoothies) equals the total grams of protein at dinner.

Women: Daily recommended protein minus the 40 grams (from the smoothies) equals the total grams of protein at dinner.

- 1 ounce of beef, chicken, or fish equals approximately 7 grams of protein
- 1 egg equals 6 grams of protein

## Example

A female requires 75 grams of protein per day. She would consume approximately 30–35 grams of protein at dinner. This is equal to approximately five or six eggs or 4–5 ounces of meat.

Need an easy way to track your macros?

There are numerous nutrition apps on the market today. I recommend downloading MyFitnessPal to your smartphone to log your food each day. It's free and easy to use, and it will give you a readout of your daily macronutrients to make sure you're staying within the 25 percent carbohydrates, 25 percent protein, and 50 percent fat ratios.

## Recommended Supplements:

- 5,000 IUs of vitamin D3 per day
- ashwagandha to help with cortisol regulation (take as directed)
- 1–2 grams (women)/2–3 grams (men) of omega-3 fatty acids to help with exercise recovery

For more information on what to order, visit the resource page at *Transformation28.net*

## The T28 Fitness Plan

- three sessions of metabolic conditioning per week for beginners

- five to six sessions of metabolic conditioning per week for accelerated results
- see appendix 1 for the T28 Challenge workouts

Each workout should be timed or scored and done at maximal intensity. Improved times or scores equal an increase in fitness. You may experience nausea after your first or second workout. This is a common, normal occurrence for those new to metabolic conditioning. It will go away after your first or second workout.

*How should I expect to feel for a few days when I start?*

- tired, lethargic
- flu-like symptoms
- mild brain fog
- irritable
- sweating
- intense sugar cravings and psychological hunger

These are normal symptoms of your body when detoxing from sugar as your insulin levels start to normalize. Be patient, and stay the course. Most people will start to feel better within three to fourteen days, depending on how unbalanced their hormones are. Don't fall for the temptation to eat sugar to help you feel better. You'll only set yourself back in the long run. Remember your big why from chapter 9.

*Note:* If you currently take medications for type 2 diabetes, it is advisable to regularly check your blood sugars. Many people often need to lower their medications within a week or two.

# CHAPTER 15

# Final Tips to Guarantee Your Success

I don't like backup plans. I like to call backup plans the "I'm planning to fail at my first plan" plan. This is not a time to have a backup plan. If you want to be successful in the T28 Challenge, you need to burn your bridges and go all in. In fact, I can tell within one day whether someone will be successful in his or her T28 Challenge by the willingness to do the following four things as soon as he or she starts:

1. *Take out the trash*: Go to your fridge, cupboards, and pantry and throw away all the junk. If it's in the house, you'll probably eat it. Why would you want it sitting there, tempting you during a moment of weakness?

2. *Have an accountability partner*: Going solo on this journey is tough. Find a friend (or your spouse) to hold you accountable to following through. Better yet, invite that person on the journey with you. Not only will it be much easier and enjoyable, but it will give you something fun to talk about. Make sure you check in with your partner every day to let him know how you're doing. Be an encouragement to her so that she can be an encouragement to you.

3. *Take your goals public*: Let as many people as possible know what you intend to do for the next twenty-eight days. Let everyone

on social media know. Take "before" and "after" pictures. Take pictures after your workouts. Take lots of pictures, and post them to social media. You'll be much less likely to fail if you have hundreds of people following you on your journey and cheering for your success.

4. *Have a war plan in place*: Failure to plan is planning to fail. Schedule your week, and take an inventory of every minute of your day. What time will you work out? What time will you eat? What time will you do your meal prep? When will you go to the grocery store? Trust me; you have plenty of time to get it done.

Doing these four things *right now* will ensure your success.

The journey to the mountaintop begins by taking that first step—and don't forget to enjoy the journey. I can't wait to see you at the mountaintop. As I and the thousands who have already done the T28 Challenge can tell you, the view is magnificent!

I can't wait to see the best version of you.

For those wanting additional resources and videos to help you on your journey, visit the "T28 Online Challenge" on the resource page at *Transformation28.net*. This course takes you step-by-step through the T28 Challenge from start to finish, and gives you all the resources to help you be successful.

# APPENDIX 1

# T28 Challenge Home Workouts Using Little to No Gym Equipment

You can find abundant video demonstrations and scaling options for each movement on my T28 Challenge online resource page. (For more information, check out the T28 Online Resources page in the back of this book.) These are additional resources for those who want additional help, guidance, and inspiration.

If you are working out three times per week, you will do all twelve of the workouts outlined below within the twenty-eight days, taking at least one rest day between workouts. If you are working out six times per week, you will repeat each workout twice, taking one rest day per week.

It is important to follow the order of the workouts exactly to allow various muscle groups adequate time to recover.

Make sure to record your score for each workout to track your improvement in fitness. You'll be amazed at how quickly you get better.

**Workout 1: Benchmark**

In seven minutes, perform the following for as many rounds and reps as possible:

- 5 burpees
- 10 air squats

Bonus round: Hold the plank position for as long as possible.

**Workout 2**

Perform as quickly as possible the following:

- 75 sit-ups
- 75 Supermans

* At the start of each minute, including the start of the workout, perform 25 jump ropes (jump-ups, singles, or double-unders).

Bonus round: Perform as many push-ups as possible in two minutes.

**Workout 3**

Perform three rounds of the following for time:

- run 400 meters
- 30 mountain climbers (right and left leg = 1 rep)

Bonus round: Hold a wall sit for as long as possible.

**Workout 4:**

Every minute on the minute for eight minutes, perform the following:

- as many air squats as possible (even minutes)
- as many push-ups as possible (odd minutes)

Bonus round: Perform an arch hold for as long as possible.

**Workout 5**

In ten minutes, perform the following for as many rounds and reps as possible:

- 25 jump ropes (jump-ups, singles, or double-unders)
- 10 mountain climbers (right and left leg = 1 rep)

Bonus round: Run 400 meters for time.

**Workout 6**

Perform five rounds of the following for time:

- 5 burpee broad jumps
- 10 sit-ups
- 15 Supermans

Bonus round: Perform as many jump ropes as possible in two minutes (jump-ups, singles, or double-unders).

**Workout 7:**

Perform three rounds of the following for time:

- run 400 meters
- 25 air squats

* Rest two minutes after each round.

Bonus round: Hold the plank position for as long as possible.

**Workout 8**

In ten minutes, perform the following for as many rounds and reps as possible:

- 2–4–6–8–10 … increasing by two reps each round until the ten minutes is up
- push-ups
- sit-ups

* Between each round, perform twenty jump ropes (jump-ups, singles, or double-unders).

Bonus round: Perform an arch hold for as long as possible.

**Workout 9**

In eight minutes, perform the following for as many rounds and reps as possible:

- 30 walking lunges (right and left leg = 2 reps)
- 15 Supermans

Bonus round: Hold a wall sit for as long as possible.

**Workout 10**

Perform the following for four rounds:

- minute 1: as many burpees as possible
- minute 2: as many jump ropes as possible (jump-ups, singles, or double-unders)
- minute 3: rest

Bonus round: Perform as many sit-ups as possible in two minutes.

**Workout 11**

Perform the following for time:
- run 400 meters
- run 800 meters
- run 400 meters

* Rest three minutes between all-out efforts.

Bonus round: Perform as many jump ropes as possible in two minutes (jump-ups, singles, or double-unders).

**Workout 12**

*Three times per week:* Perform workout 1 and bonus round, and compare your score if you are at the end of the four weeks.

*Six times per week*: Perform the following workout (if at the end of the two weeks), and begin again at workout 1 on your next workout:

In eight minutes, perform as many rounds and reps as possible of the following:

- 40 jump ropes (jump-ups, singles, or double-unders)
- 20 walking lunge steps (right and left leg = 2 reps)

Bonus round: Perform as many Supermans as possible in two minutes.

# APPENDIX 2

# The End of the T28 Challenge and the Start of Your Brand-New Life

Congratulations on finishing T28 Challenge! Let's talk about where to go from here.

*Option 1:* Choose this if you have achieved your fat-loss goals.

I recommend having a T28 smoothie in the morning and two meals per day while still adhering to all the quality foods I've outlined in this book. You can begin adding in some fruit, sweet potatoes, and legumes in moderation. Make sure to continue keeping your protein intake around .50–1.0 grams per pound of lean body mass, depending on your fitness goals.

*Option 2:* Choose this if you have not achieved your fat-loss goal and/ or you still have blood pressure, cholesterol, or blood sugar issues.

Continue on the T28 Challenge using the same protocols you used for the first twenty-eight days outlined in this book.

*Option 3*: Choose this if you have completely fallen off track and wonder what happened in six months. (You know that's not a good option, right?)

Finally, now can be the time to experiment more with your nutrition and fitness.

After completing the T28 Challenge, you can experiment with your macronutrient ratios and caloric intake. A great way to measure your success is how well you are performing your workouts. If you are feeling tired and lethargic, consider adding more fat, protein, and carbs in the proper ratios. Eventually, you'll find your sweet spot.

In addition, you also can dive into other possibilities for fueling your body. Intermittent fasting is another great eating strategy that can help calm inflammation and regenerate the immune and digestive systems. I've done this for many years on and off to help reset my body.

As your fitness improves, you'll eventually develop the need to expand your fitness routine by adding kettlebells, medicine balls, gymnastics, and barbells. I would highly recommend investing in a gym membership, where conditioning, weight training, and gymnastics are done under the watchful eye of knowledgeable coaches.

To find a gym closest to you that I recommend, visit *CrossFit.com.*

# APPENDIX 3

# Frequently Asked Questions

**Why do I feel lethargic and irritable and have a headache?**

These are symptoms of low blood sugar (hypoglycemia). Eating too many refined carbohydrates has resulted in your body not being very good at converting fat into usable energy. Give it time; let the body adapt. Within three to fourteen days, the symptoms will disappear, as will your cravings for sugar and refined carbohydrates.

**I'm taking medication for type 2 diabetes. Should I be concerned with changing my diet so drastically?**

If you're currently taking insulin or a medication to increase insulin production, you'll need to monitor your blood sugar regularly. Your insulin receptors will quickly reset themselves as you withdraw from refined carbohydrates and sugar. It is not uncommon for people to need to lower their doses of insulin or medication within five to fourteen days. Talk to your doctor about the changes that are happening. He or she should be ecstatic to help.

**Why can't I consume artificial sweeteners? Aren't they sugar-free?**

Have you ever seen a skinny (or healthy) person using artificial sweeteners? The bottom line is that all artificial sweeteners are toxic. Of all the food additives (and there are tens of thousands) available, the

FDA has received a majority of complaints about artificial sweeteners for adverse health events. Fibromyalgia, brain fog, multiple sclerosis, tumors, and increased carbohydrate cravings are all reported side effects. In fact, studies show that people who consume artificial sweeteners eat more sugar and consume more calories throughout the day, and have a higher risk for type 2 diabetes.

**Where can I purchase my food for the nutrition plan?**

You can find a majority of your food at the grocery store. You also can shop the various health food stores in your area. There are many online resources from which you can order directly. Remember, however, that not everything sold at a health food store is necessarily good for you.

**I'm craving my favorite snack. It won't hurt to eat it just this once, right?**

An addiction to sugar can be both physiological and psychological. In fact, sugar consumption elicits the same pleasurable response in the brain as nicotine, alcohol, cocaine, and heroin. Choosing to cheat will only make you crave it more and make you more likely to binge. Stay the course. It's worth it!

**I am sore after doing the workouts. Will this happen every time I work out?**

Yes and no. While you should feel sore after a workout, you should not feel pain. Keep in mind that some people need to get into better shape so that they can get into shape. After logging over two thousand high-intensity workouts over the years, I still experience soreness almost every day. When it comes to fitness, routine is the enemy, and routine will never make you sore.

**How should I feel during a workout?**

You should feel like you want to quit. If you're able to carry on a conversation during your workout, your intensity isn't high enough. The higher the intensity, the higher the release of human growth hormone (HGH). This hormone is critical for longevity, muscle building, and fat burning. Remember—not only will your body adapt to the exercise, but your mind will adapt. This will carry over in every other area of your life.

**I got on the scale today and saw that I'd gained two pounds. Yesterday I had lost five pounds. Why am I gaining weight?**

Why are you getting on the scale every day? Your body weight can fluctuate day to day by four to five pounds, depending on water retention linked to your menstrual cycle, stress, exercise, sleep, and glycogen (stored sugar) levels in muscle. Instead of focusing on the scale, focus on how your clothes fit.

**I'm not losing any weight. What gives?**

Read the previous answer, and then address this at the two- to three-week mark because some individuals are extremely weight-loss resistant. To determine your situation, you need to address these basic questions first:

- Are you doing the workouts with all-out intensity?
- Are you following the meal plan *exactly*, or are you doing your version of it?
- Are your macronutrient ratios following 25 percent/25 percent/50 percent?
- Are you avoiding fruit (remember: berries and Granny Smith apples in moderation)?

If you answered yes to all four questions, then do the following:

- Make sure you are not eating too much protein, and eat more high-fiber vegetables, preferably raw.
- Address likely toxicity issues. This can be an issue with toxicity or excess estrogen.
- Consider organic acid testing to look for underlying toxicity, gut, and stress hormone issues. This is a simple at-home test that many natural health practitioners use to help assess nutritional deficiencies at the cellular level.
- Visit a chiropractor who specializes in structural care. It may sound crazy on the surface, but spinal issues will cause an increased stress response on the brain, making it hard to lose fat.

**I don't feel like working out today, and this is getting hard. What should I do?**

Do it anyway. Yes, it is hard. If it were easy, everyone would do it. About 90 percent of the time, I'm not all that excited to work out. I do it anyway because nothing feels better than being healthy and fit for my patients, my family, and for my big why. Stay the course!

# ABOUT THE AUTHOR

Dr. Nathan Thompson is a practicing chiropractic physician in Yorkville, Illinois, who has provided the most cutting-edge natural health care in the fields of spinal correction, mobility, nutrition, and fitness since 2004. Dr. Thompson has committed his life to furthering his knowledge by attaining advanced certifications in spinal correction, nutrition, naturopathy, and CrossFit training (CF-L3). He is the creator of the revolutionary T28 Challenge that has helped thousands of people lose weight, overcome food addictions, and discover the best fitness of their lives.

In addition to practicing full-time, Dr. Thompson owns and operates CrossFit Exemplify in Morris and Yorkville, Illinois, with his wife, Barb.

He's the proud father of three future world changers: Talon, Grace, and Jacoby.

For speaking engagements and appearances, visit *Transformation28.net*.

To schedule a consultation, visit *ExemplifyHealth.com*

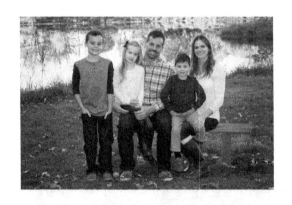

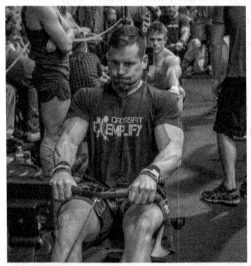

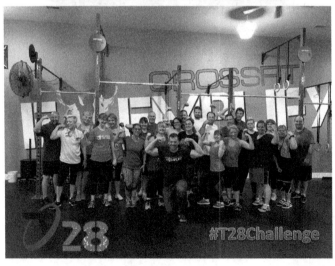

# ADDITIONAL RESOURCES

For the T28 Challenge meal plan, macronutrient calculator, and the latest nutrition and supplementation resources recommended by Dr. Nathan Thompson, visit *Transformation28.net.*

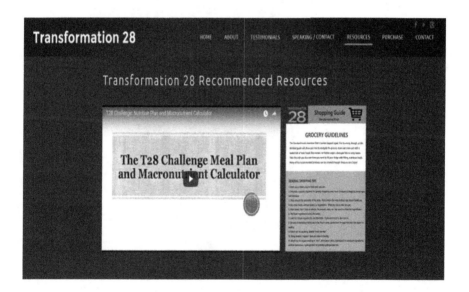

# THE T28 ONLINE CHALLENGE

Are you ready to take your T28 Challenge to the next level but don't know where to start?

Sign up for the T28 Online Challenge resources and receive the following:

- step-by-step video tutorials on how to shop, prepare, execute, and finish your T28 Challenge to ensure your success
- access to the T28 Challenge support group
- the T28 Challenge Live Nutrition Talk and *Transformation 28* e-book
- T28 Challenge–approved meal recipes and smoothie recipes and more than eighty next-level workouts
- video coaching through the twelve T28 Challenge workouts from the book
- the T28 Challenge movement vault on how to safely scale and execute all the movements from the T28 Challenge and eighty next-level workouts

Visit *Transformation28.net.*

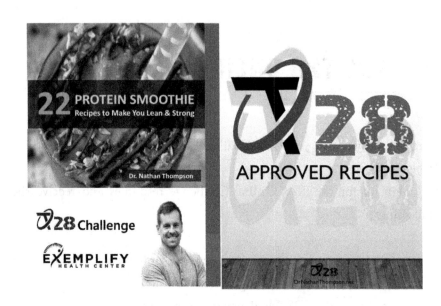

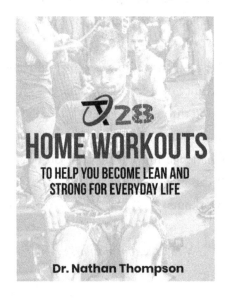

# ENDNOTES

1   "F as in Fat," *Trust for America's Health* (September 2012).

2   http://www.rwjf.org/content/dam/farm/reports/reports/2012/rwjf401318.

3   *Mayo Clinic Proceedings* 90, no. 3 (March 2015): 372–81.

4   CDC.gov.

5   Quanhe Yang, Zefeng Zhang, Edward W. Gregg et al., "Added Sugar Intake and Cardiovascular Diseases Mortality Among US Adults," *JAMA Intern Med.* (April 2014): 516–524.

6   John Carey, "Do Cholesterol Drugs Do Any Good?" *Business Week* (January 2008): 52–59.

7   http://journals.plos.org/plosone/article?id=10.1371/journal.pone.0000698.

8   *Mayo Clinic Proceedings* 90, no. 3 (March 2015): 372–81.

9   https://www.scientificamerican.com/article/widely-used-herbicide-linked-to-cancer.

10  *International Journal of Obesity and Metabolic Disorders* (2004).

11  http://www.ncbi.nlm.nih.gov/pubmed/18800291.

12  https://www.ncbi.nlm.nih.gov/pubmed/25199954.

13  http://journals.plos.org/plosone/article?id=10.1371/journal.pone.0178426.

14  https://www.ncbi.nlm.nih.gov/pmc/articles/PMC5099084/#R4.

15  Kummerow FA1, Mahfouz M, Zhou Q, Masterjohn C, "Effects of trans fats on prostacyclin production," *Scand Cardiovasc J.* (December 2013): 377–82.

16  PC Calder, "Immunoregulatory and anti-inflammatory effects of n-3 polyunsaturated fatty acids," *Brazilian Journal of Medical and Biological Research* (1998): 467–90.

17  Stoll et al. *Archives of General Psychiatry.*

18  *British Medical Journal* (October 26, 2002).

19  *New England Journal of Medicine* (April 11, 2002).

[20] F Dimeo, M Bauer, I Varahram, G Proest, and U Halter, "Benefits from aerobic exercise in patients with major depression: a pilot study," *British Journal of Sports Medicine* (April 2001): 114–17.

[21] *Journal of European Academy of Dermatology* (July 2000).

[22] H. Zhang et al., "Effect of High-Intensity Interval Training Protocol," *Kinesiology* 47, no. 1 (2015): 57–66.

[23] Pritzlaff, Wideman et al., "Catecholamine release, growth hormone secretion, and energy expenditure during exercise versus recovery in men," *J Appl Physiol* 89, no. 3 (September 2000): 937–46.

[24] R. W. Bryner, R. C. Tome, I. H. Ullrish, and R. A. Yeater, "The effects of exercise intensity on body composition, weight loss, and dietary composition in women," *J. Am. Col. Nutrition.*

[25] Dr. Arnt Erik Tjønna, *Circulation* (July 7, 2008).

[26] *Indian J Psychol Med.* 34, no. 3 (July 2012): 255–62.

[27] *Angiology* 66, no. 7 (August 2015): 613–8.

Printed in the United States
By Bookmasters